HOW TO
MEAT FREE

ECO TIPS FOR BUSY PEOPLE

STEPFANIE ROMINE

CARLTON
BOOKS

THIS IS A CARLTON BOOK

This book is 100 per cent vegan and biodegradable.

Published in 2018 by Carlton Books
An imprint of the Carlton Publishing Group
20 Mortimer Street
London W1T 3JW

Text © Carlton Books 2018
Design © Carlton Books 2018

A CIP catalogue for this book is available from the British Library.

ISBN 978-1-78739-197-0

Printed in China

10 9 8 7 6 5 4 3 2

CONTENTS

INTRODUCTION

In the past few years, we have seen a seismic shift in eating habits across Europe and North America. More and more people are opting to go meat free. Studies touting the benefits of a plant-based diet – like a healthy body weight, healthier blood pressure and blood sugar levels, and lower risks of certain cancers – are piquing the interest of those who want to live longer, healthier lives. And the compounding effects of climate change are connecting the dots between what we eat and our environmental impact. Meat comes at a price – not just a monetary one but a karmic one as well, due to the squalid conditions in which most factory-farmed animals live.

In short, the traditional meat and two veg no longer adds up for a lot of Brits. As of 2018, an estimated 7 per cent of Brits identified as vegan (and twice as many identify as vegetarian), and in the States, 6 per cent are vegan, up from 1 per cent in 2014. Elsewhere, consumers are making major shifts toward a meat-free lifestyle. For example, 44 per cent of Germans follow a "low-meat" diet. That plenty of A-list celebrities have gone vegan – Ellen DeGeneres, Moby, Beyoncé (and Jay Z), Sir Paul McCartney and Benedict Cumberbatch are all meat-free – has certainly helped the movement catch on. Even Prince Harry and Meghan Markle were reportedly eating a mostly plant-based diet leading up to their wedding.

Whether you want to give up meat for a couple of days a week, go completely vegetarian, or adapt a fully vegan diet, this book is here to make the transition easy for you. If you are making any major changes to your diet or lifestyle, please consult a healthcare professional – and always listen to your body.

HEALTHY
LIVING

Meat has long been considered the star of the plate, but the sides – vegetables, wholegrains and pulses – are now coming into the spotlight.

While meat does contain nutrients that the body needs to grow and function properly – including protein and iron – animal products are not the only source of these nutrients. Let's walk through the common nutrients you need to focus on when you give up meat and animal products.

#1
KNOW THE RISKS OF EATING MEAT – & THE BENEFITS OF NOT

Like smoking and not wearing seatbelts, eating meat – especially processed meats – is starting to fall out of fashion as we collectively become aware of the public health risks. In March 2018, the *Guardian* proclaimed, "Yes, bacon is really killing us," due to the nitrites and nitrates, which have been classified by the World Health Organization as carcinogenic alongside cigarettes, alcohol and asbestos.

A plant-based, meat-free diet can also help:

- Prevent type 2 diabetes

- Promote healthy blood pressure, thus lowering risk of heart disease and stroke

- Help you feel fuller on fewer calories, which can help control your body weight

- Lower cholesterol, due to the fibre content (which also aids regularity and healthy digestion)

- Promote clear, healthy skin, thanks to the rich antioxidant and phytochemical content of plants.

DON'T LET LABELS DEFINE YOU

"Do you" and eat a plant-based diet that suits your budget, palate and preferences. Here are some common approaches to meat-free eating, all of which can help you reap the health benefits of eating more plants:

Vegetarian: A diet that excludes meat (including poultry) and seafood, and all dishes cooked with animal-based by-products (e.g., lard and tallow, broths and stocks). Vegetarians may eat dairy and/or eggs.

Vegan: A diet that excludes all animal- and seafood-derived products (i.e. meat, poultry, seafood and related items, along with eggs, dairy, butter and even honey). This diet is often motivated by ethical or environmental concerns.

Plant-based: A meat-free diet that includes only whole, unprocessed foods. It's like a vegan diet, but plant-based eaters are often motivated by health. Plant-based and vegan are used interchangeably.

Pescatarian: A diet that excludes meat (including poultry) but includes fish and seafood.

Flexitarian: A diet that includes some animal products but is mostly vegetarian or vegan/plant based. This is a common approach to meat-free eating.

#3
TAKE IT AT YOUR OWN PACE

If a meat-free diet is new to you, don't fret over making the switch overnight. Your body will thank you each time you choose tofu bacon over a few rashers of the pork version. Every time you choose a rainbow-coloured salad at Pret A Manger over a meat pie, you're making a difference to your health. These small choices add up, and, as they feel easier and more manageable, you can add another. Whether you're giving up meat for health reasons or because you're trying to help the planet, nothing goes unnoticed.

It's also fine to indulge once in a while as you make your transition. When you're overwhelmed by a craving, sometimes it's better to give in and move on rather than let it eat away at you and stress you out. A meat-free diet should be invigorating and inspiring, not controlling or restrictive. Take it at your own pace.

#4

DON'T WORRY ABOUT WASTING AWAY

Giving up meat doesn't mean you'll wither away – on the contrary. Sports stars like Venus and Serena Williams, ultrarunner Scott Jurek and Arsenal right-back Hector Bellerin have all excelled on a meat-free diet. The U.S. Academy of Nutrition and Dietetics (AND) supports a meat-free diet for all stages of life, including during pregnancy, into older adulthood and for athletes. "Appropriately planned vegetarian, including vegan, diets are healthful, nutritionally adequate, and may provide health benefits for the prevention and treatment of certain diseases," they wrote in a 2016 position paper. Though a meat-free diet may lead to a reduced intake of certain nutrients – I'll run through these – "deficiencies can be readily avoided by appropriate planning," according to AND.

The benefits of giving up meat certainly outweigh those potential risks, especially if you put some thought into your meals and nutrition.

#5

MAINTAIN A HEALTHY WEIGHT (OR MAYBE DROP A STONE)

No matter your motivation for going meat-free, you'll reap the same health benefits. While eating less meat and more plants is always a good choice for your health and waistline, a 100 per cent meat-free, vegan diet may be the best choice for weight loss, according to a 2015 study. Researchers assigned 50 adults one of five diets – vegan, vegetarian, pescatarian, semi-vegetarian and omnivorous. Those on the vegan diet lost more than twice as much weight (7 per cent of their body weight) as those on the other diets after six months.

Whether you are trying to drop a stone or two or want to maintain your current size as you age, a plant-based diet may help.

FILL UP ON FIBRE

Fibre is only found in plants, and it's a nutrient most people in the UK are lacking, according to the British Nutrition Foundation. Though 30 grams (1.1 oz) daily is recommended, men get about 20 grams (0.7 oz) per day while women get about 17 grams (0.6 oz). Low fibre intake is linked to irregular bowel habits, as well as a higher risk of bowel cancer. However, high-fibre diets help lower cholesterol, reduce risk of diabetes, and help promote healthy body weights. Fibre comes in two forms, soluble and insoluble. Soluble fibre – found in oats, barley and legumes (beans, peas, lentils) – is sticky and forms a barrier in your gastro-intestinal (GI) tract, helping you to absorb certain nutrients and lower cholesterol. Insoluble fibre – found in vegetables and wholegrains, especially in the peels or hulls – bulks up your bowel movements to allow stool to pass through your system faster. Fibre also feeds the healthy flora of the gut and promotes healthy blood sugar levels (it slows down digestion).

#7
FILL UP ON FEWER CALORIES

Another benefit of fibre is that it slows digestion because it is indigestible. So, if you're eating meals rich in vegetables, wholegrains, legumes and fruits, you're filling your belly – and staying fuller longer – for fewer calories. Most plants are naturally lower in fat than animal products, making them less calorically dense. Carbohydrates (and protein) contain 4 calories per gram (113 calories per ounce), while fat contains more than twice that, at 9 calories per gram (255 calories per ounce).

Fibre's filling power helps promote satiety, or feelings of fullness, and helps slow digestion of fats. So, if you're one who eats with your eyes and needs to see a full plate to feel satisfied, eating more plants (and less meat) may certainly help!

If you're new to fibre, do start slow. Remember that fibre helps get things moving in your gut. Eating too much, too soon can irritate a digestive system that's used to things moving at a glacial pace. Your body will soon adjust.

KEEP CHOLESTEROL IN CHECK

Cholesterol is only found in animal products, so a meat-free diet is naturally cholesterol-free. While we usually only hear about the harm of high cholesterol levels, cholesterol does play vital roles in the body and we need it – just not too much. This waxy fat-like substance helps your body form bile acids, metabolize fat-soluble vitamins (A, D, E and K) and produce both vitamin D and steroid hormones like oestrogen and testosterone. Too much cholesterol builds up in the bloodstream, clogging arteries and interfering with blood flow.

However, a meat-free diet is associated with lower cholesterol levels, and eating more plants can help lower "bad" cholesterol (LDL, low-density lipoproteins). In addition, eating foods that contain saturated fats ("hard" or solid at room temperature) increases cholesterol levels. Animal fats, as well as tropical oils, are saturated, while eating unsaturated fats – found in plants – can help heart health and cholesterol levels, according to Heart UK.

#9

DON'T WORRY SO MUCH ABOUT PROTEIN

You'll get plenty of protein from plants! Your muscles, the brain, nervous system, skin, blood and hair are mostly protein. Amino acids, which are the building blocks of protein, play diverse roles in the body. They help us digest and metabolize food, repair our tissues, and grow and develop normally. Nine amino acids are essential, meaning our bodies can't produce them and we must get them from food.

Animal proteins are considered to be "complete" proteins, as they contain all these essential amino acids. Most plant-based proteins are called "incomplete" as they don't contain all nine (except for soya and quinoa). However, most plant-based dishes will provide a mix of amino acids (e.g. rice and beans, or a peanut butter sandwich), so as long as you eat a varied diet, you will almost certainly get all your essential amino acids.

PICK PLANTS FOR PROTEIN

With rare exceptions, every food you eat contains some protein. Plants contain a mix of macronutrients. Legumes, soya products like tofu and tempeh, nuts and seeds are common plant-based proteins, but wholegrains and vegetables provide protein, too. For example, 100 grams (3.5 oz) of cooked spinach or kale has almost 3 grams (0.1oz), while 200 grams (7 oz) of cooked brown rice has nearly 6 grams (0.2 oz). When you eat a varied meat-free diet rich in whole (unprocessed) foods, you'll get plenty of protein.

For breakfast, add seeds like hemp, chia or ground linseed to your porridge, or top with a handful of chopped nuts. Swap a tofu scramble for eggs and sausage, or toast wholemeal bread and top with nut butter and jam.

At lunch, opt for a hearty salad with veg of every colour, wholegrains like quinoa or farro, beans or peas, and nuts and seeds.

For dinner, opt for a meat-free takeaway curry, sauté tempeh with peppers and serve with brown rice, or check out the healthier, organic ready-to-eat options at your local supermarket.

#11
DON'T FORGET ABOUT IRON

Iron is an essential mineral that regulates cell growth. It also supports the immune system (by boosting resistance to stress and disease) and the production of haemoglobin, which transports oxygen from the lungs to your tissues and carbon dioxide back to the lungs. Women of child-bearing age are more at risk of being iron deficient (due to blood loss from menstruation), but since iron can build up in the body, confirm any suspected deficiencies with your GP before supplementing.

PUMP UP THE (NON-HEME) IRON

While it's true that red meat provides iron, there are plenty of other sources – and without all the saturated fat and cholesterol! Iron that comes from animal and seafood sources is called heme iron, while plant-based and supplemental sources are known as non-heme. Plant-based sources of iron include blackstrap molasses, fortified cereals, dark chocolate, lentils, pulses (white beans, kidney beans, chickpeas and peas), potatoes and nuts.

- Drizzle molasses on your morning porridge, use it in baked goods and add to sauces for a complex subtle sweetness.

- Savour your chocolate – 85 grams (3 oz) of 70–85 per cent cocoa-solid dark chocolate provides 10 milligrams of iron, 67 per cent of a woman's recommended daily value and more than 100 per cent of a man's.

- Cook your food in cast-iron pans. When well-seasoned, you won't need to use added oils.

- Combine iron-rich foods with vitamin C, which can boost absorption. Drizzle lemon juice on spinach, add tomatoes to your pulses, or eat bell peppers alongside your potatoes.

#13

KNOW YOUR BONES NEED MORE THAN CALCIUM

We've been told since we were tots that drinking milk builds strong bones. The most abundant mineral in our bodies, calcium helps build strong bones, teeth and muscle tissue. It also triggers muscle contractions, regulates your heartbeat and nerve function and aids blood clotting.

Though calcium is usually touted as the mineral responsible for strong, healthy bones, it doesn't work alone. With regard to bone health, calcium works in conjunction with vitamins D and K, and magnesium. Vitamin D helps the body absorb calcium from food, vitamin K aids bone metabolism (and may protect against osteoporosis) and magnesium aids mineralization of bones.

On a plant-based diet, without dairy, there are plenty of other ways to meet your calcium needs.

FIND DAIRY-FREE
CALCIUM SOURCES

With the exception of vitamin D (more on that later), you can get all those nutrients from plants. Calcium is found in all plants, but greens like mustard or turnip greens, kale, bok choy, collards and watercress all contain the highest, most bioavailable amounts.

Many plant-based milks are calcium-fortified and tofu often contains it as well (calcium is used as a coagulant). Almonds, tahini, figs, oranges and white beans also contain some calcium.

- Use fortified non-dairy milks in place of cow's milk.

- Swap tahini for oils in your salad dressing.

- Snack on almonds and figs, or add them to salads and Buddha bowls.

- Eat your greens. Finely chop them and stir into soups and stews. Sauté or steam and drizzle with balsamic and tahini. Add calcium-rich greens to your usual salad greens.

#15
BE MINDFUL ABOUT B VITAMINS

Vitamin B12 is not found in plants, but it is found in meat, eggs, milk products and seafood. When you stop eating those foods, you need to seek out other sources of this essential vitamin. B12 is responsible for cell development, nervous system function and metabolism of fat and protein. As a water-soluble vitamin, B12 is not stored in the body; excess is excreted through the urine. Low levels can cause nervous system issues and anaemia. Consider supplementing but talk to your GP first. As long as you consume fortified foods or supplements, you are actually less likely to suffer B12 deficiency than a meat eater, according to the Vegan Society.

You can get B12 via a meat-free diet from fortified foods like breakfast cereals and non-dairy milks. Check the label to see whether a food contains added B12. Nutritional yeast (see p.43) is also fortified with B12.

MIND YOUR MINERALS

In addition to calcium, two minerals that can be lacking in a meat-free diet are zinc and iodine. Zinc is found in meat, liver, eggs and seafood – as well as wholegrains – and it plays a role in digestion and metabolism. Zinc also plays a role in reproductive-system development and helps with healing. To get zinc from a meat-free diet, include plenty of soya products, legumes, grains, cheese, seeds and nuts, or discuss supplements with your GP. Iodine is found in iodized salt and seafood, as well as sea vegetables. This mineral plays an important role in thyroid health. Consider using iodized salt, taking supplements and including a wide range of seaweed, like nori, dulse and kelp, in your daily diet. Artisan salts – including pink Himalayan – and salt condiments like miso and tamari are often not iodized.

#17
DO MONITOR YOUR VITAMIN D

Vitamin D plays a vital role in forming healthy teeth and bones, and it helps the heart and nervous system function, too. Though it's called the "sunshine vitamin" because our bodies can metabolize vitamin D from sunlight, during winter or living at higher latitudes means you might not get enough. Meat eaters get D from liver, egg yolks, the cream in butter and fortified milk. If you're forgoing meat, you'll need to get it from fortified sources, including mushrooms that have been exposed to UV light and fortified non-dairy milks. Or talk to your doctor about taking a supplement.

#18
DON'T OVERLOOK OMEGA-3 FATTY ACIDS

The essential fatty acids known as omega-3s have been touted in recent years for their role in supporting brain and heart health. Found in fatty fish (like salmon and tuna), nuts, linseed, chia seeds and some vegetable oils, there are actually three types of omega-3s: eicosapentaenoic acid (EPA), docosahexaenoic acid (DHA) and alpha-linolenic acid (ALA). ALA is the only one that's truly essential and it's also the most common one in our diet. EPA, which is strongly linked to fighting inflammation, and DHA, which is linked to mental health, come primarily from fish; ALA comes mostly from plant foods. While we can convert ALA to the other two, studies have shown that we don't convert it efficiently. In addition to including plant-based foods that contain omega-3s, like nuts, seeds and leafy greens, consider adding algae oil or vegan omega-3 supplements to your diet, under the supervision of your GP.

#19
GET FAMILIAR WITH PHYTOCHEMICALS

Phytochemicals are simply chemicals in plants that provide scent, colour and flavour – and nutritional benefits when you consume them. Many of them act as antioxidants, neutralizing free radicals that can cause inflammatory responses in the body. These substances support your immune system, protect your DNA and cells, promote healthy cell development and turnover and prevent harmful substances in our food and drink from becoming carcinogenic, according to the American Institute for Cancer Research.

You may have heard the advice to "eat the rainbow" and these phytonutrients are responsible for the vibrant hues found in plants. Each colour is responsible for a different phytonutrient, with its own distinct role in supporting your health. There's no need to memorize the lengthy, scientific names – simply eat an array of different coloured plants daily! Eating in Technicolor is a fun, delicious way to reap the benefits of a meat-free diet.

DON'T LET IT STRESS YOU OUT!

If you don't know vitamin A from zinc and haven't counted a gram or ounce of protein in your life, you can still enjoy a healthy meat-free diet. As long as you eat a variety of plants daily and limit your consumption of processed, salty and sugary foods, you'll have a healthy diet. Check in with your GP before making any major changes to your diet.

In addition to learning about the health benefits of adopting this approach, I'll explain in the remaining chapters how to ensure you maintain a balanced diet. I'll share a comprehensive list of meat-free alternatives and staples for your cupboard and walk you through all possible scenarios of a meat-free life: dining out, eating with friends and getting creative in the kitchen. These tips will help you lead a plant-based, meat-free life.

SURVIVING WITHOUT MEAT

I have a friend, Hannah, who likes to use the hashtag #anythingyoucaneaticaneatvegan. And it's true. If you haven't ventured into the vegetarian section of your supermarket lately, there's a lot more out there than tofu and beans. From bacon rashers and bangers, burgers and mince to fried chicken and pulled pork, it's true that there is now a meat-free alternative to every food you can think of.

#21
IDENTIFY YOUR EXISTING MEAT-FREE OPTIONS

Before you start worrying about all the time and effort you'll need to put forth to learn to cook without meat, reflect on your favourite meals. You've probably eaten plenty of meat-free and vegan meals, appetizers and snacks without thinking about it.

Some of your favourite comfort foods and treats may be 100 per cent meat-free: bean burritos, hummus (or baba ganoush) and pitta bread, sourdough bread with olive oil and balsamic, cucumber or avocado rolls, spring rolls, peanut butter (and jam) sandwiches, spaghetti and marinara sauce, chips (with vinegar or ketchup!), jacket potatoes, crisps (most of them), garden salads with vinaigrette, soft pretzels with mustard and tortilla chips with salsa (and guacamole). You likely eat vegetables and/or fruit at most meals, too.

While many of these aren't foods you should be eating daily (ahem, chips and crisps!), the above list contains reliable meat-free options you can cook already or find in most restaurants.

START WITH PULSES

Pulses might not satisfy your craving for a steak (though plenty of meat-free options abound for such a hankering), but they are a nutritious, affordable, tasty staple. Whether you buy them tinned or cook dried ones at home, pulses are versatile and packed with protein, fibre and other nutrients.

Drain and rinse tinned beans to reduce sodium and ease digestion. If beans and lentils cause bloating for you, just keep eating them. The more often you eat beans, the more acclimatized your body will become to them and the more your body will produce the enzyme needed to digest them, reducing gas.

- Lentils are the fastest-cooking legume, making them ideal for busy weeknight dinners. Pair them with spicy sauces or atop jacket potatoes.

- Chickpeas are lovely in salads and wraps, while I like creamy white beans – blended or whole – in pasta sauce.

- Add black and pinto beans to burritos and tacos, and use split peas for slow-cooked dishes.

#23
SATISFY BEEFY CRAVINGS WITH SEITAN

Seitan is concentrated wheat gluten, and once cooked and seasoned, it has a taste and texture that's similar to meat. While obviously off-limits for those with coeliac disease, seitan makes juicy and hearty steaks, roasts and burgers. You can find powdered vital wheat gluten alongside flour, to season and customize to your liking, and ready-made seitan products are commonly available these days.

Seitan is a rather heavy food, so I eat it sparingly – use it as you would red meat, actually. If it's new to you, start with a small amount. Seitan can tolerate long cooking times and marinades, so you can dice it for braises or stews, or keep it whole for a meat-free roast.

- Thinly slice marinated seitan, then sear as you would flank steak. Serve on a roll with rocket, basil, mayonnaise and thinly sliced red onion.

- Dice, shred or slice seitan and cook with barbecue sauce or fajita spices. Wrap in a tortilla with greens and guacamole.

- Season and braise seitan in place of short ribs, Korean BBQ or carne asada.

#24
TRY TEMPEH

Tempeh is a fermented soya protein native to Indonesia. Soya beans are cooked, then inoculated and allowed to ferment. The fermentation process breaks down the soya to make it more digestible. The result is a firm yet spongy protein that can be marinated, sautéed or fried. Tempeh has a slight bitterness that steaming will remove and it's delightful sauced. Since it has a stronger flavour than tofu, pair it with bold flavours and traditional ones (like HP Sauce).

- Grate, cube or crumble tempeh, then brown it as you would mince. Season to taste for taco filling, bolognese, lasagne or chilli.

- Steamed cubed tempeh can stand in for chicken in bound salads – substitute mashed avocado for the mayo if you prefer.

- Thinly slice tempeh, then marinate as desired – try 60 ml (2 fl oz) of rice vinegar, 1 tablespoon of tamari, 1 tablespoon of toasted sesame oil, chilli flakes to taste and a few minced cloves of garlic. Drain and pan-fry until browned. Mix any leftover marinade with 125 ml (4 fl oz) of water and bring to a boil, then simmer until thickened.

#25

GIVE TOFU ANOTHER TRY

If you find tofu to be bland and squishy, you're not alone – when not prepared or seasoned properly, it doesn't have much character. However, I like to think of it as a blank canvas.

There are two basic forms: soft and firm. Soft tofu is best used in smoothies, scrambles (in place of eggs) or soups. Once drained and pressed to remove excess water, firm tofu can be used in just about any recipe that calls for chicken or poultry. (The easiest way to press tofu is to place a block on a cutting board between tea towels, then place a heavy pot on top for about 10 minutes.)

Thin slices of tofu can be pan-seared and used in chicken dishes like marsala, piccata or cacciatore. Or season it and coat in breadcrumbs for a meat-free schnitzel.

For an even chewier texture, freeze tofu, then thaw it and squeeze out excess water.

#26
MAKE MUSHROOMS A MAIN DISH

We tend to consider mushrooms to be a side dish or ingredient, but these fungi are packed with protein, fibre and – depending on the variety – nutrients like vitamin D, potassium and antioxidants.

Mushrooms contain the amino acid glutamate, which provides the flavour known as umami (a Japanese word meaning "pleasant savoury taste"), and they add depth and richness to meat-free dishes.

To maximize their flavour in any dish, start by browning your mushrooms, which releases their deep, earthy deliciousness, along with your aromatics, herbs and spices. (If you're not a fan of the texture, use a food processor to mince them first.)

Every week, sauté a diced onion or a few shallots with 150 grams (5 oz) of sliced or diced mushrooms, plus fresh herbs, garlic and a glug or two of dry white wine or sherry. Season with salt and pepper, and use as the basis for quick meals – with steamed grains, sautéed veg or simple tofu or legumes.

MIX UP YOUR MUSHROOMS

Here are a few common mushrooms you can use in place of meat.

King oysters: These large, mild-tasting mushrooms can be shredded in place of pulled pork or chicken, sliced crosswise to stand in for scallops, or thickly cut lengthwise as a mild whitefish swap.

Oysters: These delicate, nutrient-rich mushrooms are delicious seared in a hot cast-iron pan, with a simple white wine sauce. They can also be broken into "petals" and browned, then added to soups and stews.

Boletes and buttons: These are the workhorses of the mushroom world. Use them in any dish to add flavour and nutrition. Boletes are especially good diced in Bolognese pasta sauce.

Shiitake, maitake and bunapi: These Asian mushrooms can be thinly sliced or broken into small clumps and added to stir-fries. Shiitakes are especially rich in umami, so add a couple of dried caps (broken into pieces) to any dish that would normally use beef or lamb.

#28
GO NUTS

Nuts and seeds are calorically dense, and they're high in protein, fibre, B vitamins and some minerals. They also contain omega-3 fatty acids, which are good for heart and brain health.

- Add nut butter to smoothies to give them staying power, or use in place of oil in salad dressings. Drizzle peanut or almond butter sauces over steamed vegetables and brown rice.

- Top salads with chopped, roasted hazelnuts, walnuts and pecans.

- Stir chopped nuts or seeds into cooked grains, along with fresh herbs, dried fruit and an acid like lemon juice or cider vinegar, for a quick meal.

- Snack on a handful of nuts and seeds.

- Soak raw cashews and blend with water, then season to taste with lemon juice and salt for a rich, dairy-free cream. (Start with 1½ parts water to 1 part cashews.)

- Add hemp and sesame seeds to salads or stir-fries.

#29

GET CREATIVE WITH JACKFRUIT

This tropical fruit is sweet when ripe, but while it's green, it has very little flavour and can be used as a stringy meat substitute. Look for whole jackfruit or canned green jackfruit at Asian markets. Use it in place of tuna or crab in any recipe, or toss with enchilada or mole sauce.

Pre-seasoned jackfruit is popping up in the refrigerated pseudo-meat section of supermarkets. Try Thai curry, BBQ or sriracha flavours.

If you prefer to cook from scratch, drain and rinse canned jackfruit, then marinate it for at least a couple of hours. Drain excess marinade before sautéing.

#30

EMBRACE CHICKPEA FLOUR

Also known as garbanzo beans (or gram/besan) flour, this gluten-free flour is used in cuisines from Southeast Asia to northern Africa and southern Europe. In Myanmar, chickpea flour is cooked like a porridge, cooled and cubed, then prepared like tofu. In Ethiopia, it's a main ingredient in shiro wat, a creamy stew seasoned with berbere, a traditional spice mix. And across southern France, you can wash down your delicious socca (chickpea flour pancakes) with a glass of crisp rosé.

Always cook your chickpea flour thoroughly – it should never be doughy in the centre. Since chickpea flour is made from ground, dried chickpeas, it can cause bloating and GI upset if not completely cooked.

RECIPE: SOCCA

Socca is a satisfying, simple savoury dish. Here's how to make your own:

Mix 250 ml (8.5 fl oz) each of water and chickpea flour, along with 60 ml (2 fl oz) of olive oil. Add ¾ teaspoon of salt, plenty of black pepper and (optional) ½ teaspoon of ground turmeric. You can also stir in chopped herbs and shallots. Let sit for 30 minutes and preheat your grill. Heat a cast-iron frying pan on the stove. Add the batter, cook for two minutes, covered, then uncover and transfer to the grill for 8-10 minutes, until the edges are crisp and the top is nice and brown. Serve immediately, with a rocket salad on top.

#31

FOR QUICK MEALS,
COOK UP QUINOA

Truly a pseudo cereal versus a whole grain, quinoa is a complete protein, which is rare for plants. It cooks in 10 or so minutes once your water starts to boil, making it perfect for busy week nights. Pair with your favourite vegetable and a sauce for a balanced meal.

- Swap quinoa for your morning oats. Top with fruit and a bit of maple syrup or cashew cream.

- Toss cooled quinoa with greens and a shallot vinaigrette for a simple yet elegant salad.

- Serve in place of pasta, especially with hearty sauces like mushroom Bolognese.

SPRINKLE NUTRITIONAL YEAST ON EVERYTHING

Nutritional yeast is a staple for vegans. Not only does it add protein, fibre and B vitamins to any dish, it also has a delicious, cheesy taste. Nooch, as it's known, is a versatile, nutrient-rich ingredient. I keep a small shaker bottle of it in my handbag when I travel.

- Sprinkle nooch liberally over pasta, vegetables or salads.

- Shake it on pizza if you're skipping the cheese.

- Mix into salsa, hummus or tomato sauce.

- Add to veggie wraps and sandwiches.

- Stir a spoonful into soup.

- Combine with almond meal, salt and garlic powder for a quick vegan parmesan swap.

- Use it on air-popped popcorn with olive oil, salt and pepper, plus chilli flakes if you like heat.

START SMALL AND EASE INTO IT, IF YOU WANT

Some people go meat free overnight, while others gradually phase out animal products. However you choose to change your habits is up to you – there's no "wrong" way. As a health coach with training in behavioural science, I encourage clients to take all goals one step at a time. Once a habit feels manageable, add another. This creates lasting change.

To maintain your motivation toward a meat-free, vegan or vegetarian diet or lifestyle, look within for inspiration. Threats, rewards and punishments – all forms of extrinsic motivation – don't motivate us in the long run. What works best is intrinsic motivation, which comes from within. With intrinsic motivation, you want to change because you genuinely are interested in doing so and you find your new habit or behaviour to be fun or pleasant. Identifying as a meat-free eater, vegan or vegetarian can also help you stay motivated by making it a part of your personality or belief system.

#34
GET CREATIVE WITH VEGGIE BURGERS

In my 12 years of meat-free living, I've lost count of how many veggie burgers I've eaten. They're an easy option for restaurants to have on the menu for meat-free eaters, so you're going to encounter a lot of them. Here's what you should know.

Veggie burgers can run the gamut from healthy fare to junk food and from delicious to, well, barely passable. Homemade ones can be as nutrient dense as you'd like them to be, made with legumes and plenty of vegetables, herbs and spices. Store-bought ones have come a long way, but many contain processed soy and more salt and fat than is necessary. Read the labels and avoid any that contain ingredients you don't recognize.

As with meat-based ones, the real fun comes in topping your veggie burgers. Beyond traditional condiments, I love using avocado, sprouts, salsa, chutney or even hummus. I share a simple recipe for veggie burgers on p.113.

#35
KEEP ENJOYING SUNDAY ROAST

I grew up eating roast beef or ham every Sunday with my extended family. While the meat was at the centre of the table, there were plenty of meat-free options, too. Mashed potatoes, green beans and a large salad were always present, plus fresh yeasted rolls and other veggie sides. These days, when I join my loved ones for a holiday feast, I avoid the meat but still have plenty to eat.

Maintain your traditional weekly meal by simply leaving out the meat and ramping up the veg. In place of a roasted joint, you could make a homemade seitan version (pp.32–3), substitute meat with mushrooms – which are just as rich and tasty as meat! – or serve a legume dish on the side. Use the meaty marinade on p.103 to infuse your roast vegetables with umami, and swap meat for mushrooms in your onion gravy.

CHUCK YOUR CHICKEN, BUT ENJOY YOUR FAVOURITE DISHES

My mom's go-to dish was always chicken – chicken piccata, chicken stir-fry, crunchy baked chicken, chicken paprikash... you get the picture. Most of my favourite childhood dishes involved chicken, but I found it easy to swap the chicken in those dishes for a meat-free ingredient instead. Here are some suggestions.

- Season tofu or tempeh with poultry seasoning (sage, thyme, marjoram, rosemary, nutmeg, salt and black pepper).

- Swap chickpeas for chicken in stews and soups.

- Use Quorn (often contains egg whites) or another premade meat-free fillet.

- For homemade "chick-un" nuggets, marinate tofu or tempeh, then bread and bake as desired.

- For stir-fries, curries and other such dishes, use chickpeas, tofu or tempeh.

- Mix puréed white beans or chickpeas into homemade seitan along with poultry seasoning.

#37
LET STIR-FRIES BECOME A STAPLE

Even without a designated meat replacement, stir-fries are an easy, filling vegan dish. By serving them with brown rice or another whole grain (instead of processed white rice), you're adding another source of protein.

Get creative: Use a rainbow of vegetables, from the routine ones like onions, peppers and carrots to more unusual ones like bamboo shoots, baby corn and lotus root. Aubergine, courgettes and broccoli are also good additions to a stir-fry.

Start your stir-fry with cubed tofu and tempeh if you want more protein, or shake on sesame seeds and sliced and toasted almonds before serving.

Keep your seasoning simple with a combination of rice vinegar, soy sauce and toasted sesame oil, as well as other umami-rich additions like fermented black beans, hoisin sauce (check whether it contains fish sauce), miso paste or chilli flakes.

COUNT ON CURRIES

While the list of herbs and spices needed to make an authentic curry might be intimidating, the resulting rich flavour is worth it. Curries are the backbone of my meat-free menus. I make them with tofu, tempeh and legumes, or sometimes just a mixture of fresh veggies.

If you're truly overwhelmed by the idea of cooking up a curry, start with a spice blend or sauce from the supermarket. Or try this simple version:

RECIPE:

Begin with a tin of full-fat coconut milk. Drain the water into a cup, then put the solids into a pan. Heat until melted, then add a generous amount of yellow curry powder, grated ginger and minced garlic. Heat until fragrant, stirring often. Add onions and sauté until soft, then add veggies of choice, a drained and rinsed tin of chickpeas and the coconut water. Add a cup or two of veg broth, cover and simmer until tender. Season to taste with salt and lime juice.

#39

BE INVENTIVE WITH SAVOURY PIES

Shepherd's or cottage pie is just as tasty without the meat. Savoury pies are, too. It's quite simple to make meat-free versions of these traditional comfort foods.

- Swap vegan butter or olive oil and non-dairy milk (try the cashew option on p.111) in the potato topping on your shepherd's pie to make it vegan.

- Likewise, use olive oil or vegan butter in your pie dough.

- Use lentils and mushrooms in place of mince – or try one of the readymade plant-based mince products if you prefer a more authentic taste and texture.

- Vegemite and dark miso paste are my secret ingredients for adding meaty flavour to veg dishes. Both are packed with umami!

- Puff pastry usually contains butter, but filo dough does not. You can use a light spray of olive or another oil between layers in place of butter.

UPGRADE YOUR SANDWICHES

Though the headline focused on bacon, deli slices and other processed meats are also part of the WHO analysis of carcinogens in meats. If you're accustomed to ordering a ham and cheese or club sandwich for lunch, you might feel at a loss when it comes to delis but there are plenty of meat-free sandwiches to enjoy.

- Avocado toast, while not a traditional sandwich, is a satisfying meat-free swap, especially when drizzled with balsamic and topped with rocket or sprouts, plus a sprinkling of sea salt.

- Hummus makes a wonderful sandwich spread. Add olives, roasted red peppers, rocket or spinach and thin slices of cucumber and red onion.

- Don't forget falafel! While not a sandwich per se, it is a tasty, meat-free option in wraps and flatbreads.

- If you don't consume dairy or eggs, opt for avocado or hummus in place of mayonnaise or creamy dressings and sauces.

SAVING MONEY

Meat, seafood and dairy are usually the most expensive categories of food, so transitioning to a vegetarian or vegan diet can be a good way to save your pennies. However, to ensure your meals are healthy and flavourful, you might need to stock your pantry and fridge with some new-to-you ingredients. But you don't need to break the bank to build a meat-free kitchen. Here are ways of keeping your diet exciting while also keeping an eye on your purse strings.

#41

STOP BUYING MEAT & DAIRY

While this tip might seem obvious, given the title of this book, I'd like to remind you that you're saving money simply by going meat free. A 2015 study in the *Journal of Hunger & Environmental Nutrition* compared a plant-based diet to an omnivorous one recommended by the US government. The "MyPlate" plan cost an extra $750 (about £550 or $991 AUS) per year with fewer servings of vegetables, fruits and wholegrains!

When I gave up meat, fish and dairy, my grocery bills were much smaller, which allowed me to divert money to things like herbs and spices or kitchen equipment.

You'll also save money when dining out, as meat-based main dishes are almost always more costly than vegetarian or vegan ones (more on that in Going Out, pp.74–95). While it's likely that your bottom line wasn't the reason you gave up meat (or are considering it), it's definitely a nice side effect.

BUY IN BULK

Bulk bins are common in supermarkets in the US; from curry powder to oats, pinto beans to raw almonds, you can buy almost any unprocessed ingredient in bulk, meaning you can buy as much or as little of an ingredient as you'd like. In the UK, Whole Foods Market and some other grocery stores are starting to add bulk bins. When you buy food in this way, you're not paying for packaging, marketing, or other expenses. You're getting food, plain and simple. When you're making a dish that calls for six new-to-you spices or you want to try a couple of different types of gluten-free flour, head to the bulk section and buy just as much as you need – and keep some extra cash in your pocket. I buy everything from grains and beans to spices and nuts in bulk.

Tip: Save money on pricey snacks, and mix together a few different types of bulk nuts, seeds and dried fruit – plus some chocolate chips.

#43

EAT WHOLE FOODS

Processing foods not only adds unwanted fat, sugars and salt, but it also drives up the price. To save money, eat what nature provides, then prepare and season it yourself. This keeps you in control of what's in your food and it can help you stick to a budget too. Beyond fruits and vegetables, choose plain wholegrains and legumes. Tinned beans are budget-friendly, but dried ones are even more so. Anything that is pre-cooked, pre-seasoned or prepared will cost more. While it's fine to occasionally choose time over money and opt for convenience foods, your meat-free diet will be healthier and more affordable if you cook from scratch as often as you're able.

#44

CHOOSE FOODS IN SEASON

Thanks to globalization, we can enjoy most fruits and vegetables year round – but it comes at a price. Your carbon footprint aside, the sticker price on out-of-season produce will be higher than that growing right here, right now. Fruit and veggies also just taste better when they are in season and allowed to ripen naturally.

Here are some examples of seasonal foods:

Winter: apples, beetroot, Brussels sprouts, cabbage, carrots, celery, kale, leeks, onions, parsnips, spring greens, spring onions, squash, swedes, turnips, winter squash.

Spring: artichoke, asparagus, aubergine, beetroot, cucumber, elderflowers, lettuce, peas, peppers, potatoes, radishes, rhubarb, rocket, spinach, spring onions, watercress.

Summer: aubergine, beetroot, blackberries, blueberries, broad beans, broccoli, carrots, cauliflower, cherries, courgettes, cucumber, currants, fennel, garlic, gooseberries, onions, peas, potatoes, radishes, raspberries, rocket, runner beans, strawberries, summer squash, swiss chard, tomatoes, turnips, watercress, watermelon.

Autumn: aubergine, beetroot, broccoli, Brussels sprouts, butternut squash, carrots, cauliflower, celery, courgettes, cucumber, garlic, kale, kohlrabi, leeks, lettuce, onions, parsnips, pears, peppers, plums, potatoes, pumpkin, radishes, rhubarb, rocket, runner beans, spinach, swiss chard, turnips, watercress.

#45

COOK BIGGER BATCHES

Let "cook once, eat twice" (or thrice!) become your motto. While it might take an hour to prepare a recipe, it won't take two hours to make a double batch of that recipe. You'll likely not even notice the extra few minutes of work, but you will notice that you don't have to make dinner or lunch the next day!

I employ this tactic for staples like quinoa and brown rice, roasted vegetables and tofu scramble, so I can add the extra portions to quick meals throughout the week. You can easily double up recipes like stir-fries, soups and stews. I skip this tip for overly fussy recipes or those that are delicate – such as any dish that has a crisp crust, or contains fresh herbs or delicate greens that spoil quickly.

PLAN YOUR MEALS

It might seem like a tedious chore, but if you want to stick to a food budget, you need to plan ahead. Making a shopping list is a good first step toward reducing impulse purchases. Take it one step further: know which meals you'll eat on which day for the coming week or couple of days. This eliminates the need to run to the store every day, except for perishables, and it will help reduce food waste. A third of the food produced for humans to consume is wasted, so every bit helps. If you don't like the rigidity of planning meals far in advance, start with a couple of dinners a week. Or, if you're in the habit of buying pricey smoothies en route to the office instead of making breakfast at home, perhaps you could commit to a week of preparing your morning meals for yourself.

#47

JOIN A WAREHOUSE CLUB

Costco and other members-only clubs carry plenty of meat-free staples at lower prices. Here's how you can use a warehouse club to save on meat-free foods.

- Steer clear of the crisps and processed snacks, and reach for the basics. Load up on nuts, dried fruit, quinoa and other grains, spices, olive oil, tinned tomatoes and beans, non-dairy milk, flour and sugar, seaweed, frozen fruits and vegetables.

- I sometimes splurge on a case of green juices or kombucha (fermented tea drink), as it is far cheaper than buying them one at a time.

- Only buy what you know you can consume before it goes stale or spoils. Transfer surplus ingredients to sealed containers to prolong shelf life.

- Keep an eye out for deals on kitchen appliances, like high-speed blenders, juicers and air fryers.

- If you have a small household, consider splitting the membership and purchases with a friend.

PERFECT A FEW SIMPLE RECIPES

The adage "walk before you run" holds true in the kitchen, especially as you're adapting to a new way of eating. Bypass the complicated recipes and start with the basics. Try lasagne with tofu ricotta, a tempeh stir-fry or grilled mushroom kebabs. Getting Creative, pp.96–117, contains some simple recipes that can help you get started.

- Make a goal of trying one new recipe every week or so, adding to your repertoire as you gain confidence.

- Be sure to follow recipes to the letter when you're starting out, especially if they contain ingredients that are new to you.

- Set yourself up to succeed by starting with techniques that you already know, such as sautéing or roasting.

- Get comfortable with a knife. If you eat a meat-free diet,you're going to need to know how to prepare vegetables, and you'll need a good, sharp knife to do so. Dull knives are more dangerous than sharp ones, so keep yours sharp and know where your fingers are at all times!

#49

STRATEGIZE YOUR ORGANIC AND CONVENTIONAL PURCHASES

Organic produce isn't more nutritious than conventionally grown produce, but it is lower in additional toxins than our bodies have to process. Organic options are pricier but worth the cost if you can afford them. As much as I would love to buy 100 per cent organic foods, I can't always find or afford them. These tips can help you prioritize which foods to buy organic.

- The more delicate a vegetable, fruit or herb, the more likely it is to absorb pesticides. Opt for organic salad greens, berries and fresh herbs like basil and parsley.

- You can choose conventional versions of thick-skinned foods like avocados, pineapple and melons. However, wash the exterior thoroughly before cutting into them.

- Remove the peels and outer leaves of conventional produce to reduce exposure.

- Keep an eye out for deals on kitchen appliances, like high-speed blenders, juicers, and air fryers.

- For more info about choosing organic versus conventional based on pesticides, look up the Environmental Working Group, Food Standards Agency or your local equivalent.

LEARN TO DIY

Everything comes with a cost, be it time, energy, know-how or actual currency. If you have time and are willing to learn, making foods from scratch versus buying them from the store will help you save a lot. Veggie burgers (start with the recipe on p.113), almond milk, coconut yogurt and cashew cheese are all foods I used to buy but now make. In addition, I make granola, pasta sauces, bread (sometimes) and pizza dough. While not all of these foods are special to a meat-free diet, they are cheaper, regardless.

There's a certain satisfaction that comes from making something you thought impossible, like a perfect loaf of sourdough that's crisp on the outside, soft and pillowy on the inside. If you're hesitant, invite a friend over and open a bottle of wine or make tea while you make it. You'll either gain a new skill or have a good story!

#51
STREAMLINE YOUR MEALS

Resist falling into the comparison trap when you see other people's meat-free meals on Instagram. As beautiful and inspiring as those bloggers' and influencers' meals may be, that's not how most of us eat on a daily basis.

Keep your meals simple and follow this formula

- A protein: tofu, tempeh, legumes, veggie burger, quinoa, etc.

- A grain or starchy vegetable: brown rice, wholemeal pasta, farro, freekeh, spelt, potatoes, sweet potatoes, beetroots, etc.

- Two non-starchy veg: make one of them green.

- A sauce or seasoning.

Some sample meals might be:

- A jacket potato with beans, spinach and a spicy slaw.

- A tempeh stir-fry with brown rice, kale, peppers and tamari.

- A veggie burger on a wholemeal bun (your choice of toppings), with a salad of watercress and cherry tomatoes.

#52

KNOW WHEN TO SPLURGE AND WHEN TO SAVE

When you buy name-brand foods, you pay extra for the marketing, advertising, etc. Store brands are usually almost identical in quality (and sometimes superior) but cost far less.

Reach for the store-brand version of staple items like tinned tomatoes and beans, frozen fruit or vegetables, pasta, wholegrains, flour and other dry ingredients.

Spend more on any item to which you have brand loyalty – perhaps it's a special type of salsa or chutney. If you're attached to that particular flavour, anything else will fall short and disappoint you.

Many stores are investing in their own brands and offering more premium products – both processed and not – at a lower cost than name brands. For example, Tesco hired Derek Sarno, formerly global chef at Whole Foods Market, to be their chef director of plant-based innovation. Launched in 2017, the Wicked Kitchen line offers meat-free (100 per cent vegan, to be specific) meals and dishes that are healthy and nutritious.

#53

FOCUS ON PLANTS, PLAIN AND SIMPLE

You don't need superfoods, protein powders or trendy meat analogues. You might want them, but your meat-free diet will get on quite nicely without them.

To save money, emphasize whole foods at every meal. Fill half of your plate with vegetables in as many colours as you can manage. Fill the rest of your plate with other plants – fruits, legumes, grains, nuts and seeds, etc. – and you'll be eating as Mother Nature intended!

There's a trick to avoiding junk food and saving money at grocery stores, and it can apply even if the supermarkets where you live are set up a bit differently. Shop the perimeter! The good stuff is more often than not placed around the edges of the store, while the processed snacks are in the middle aisles. Avoid those, and you've resisted the unhealthy stuff. I also bypass the entire dairy aisle and meat and fish departments, too.

#54
GROW YOUR OWN

I'm not suggesting you give up your flat and buy a farm in the country. Grow what you can based on your home. Plant blueberry bushes in your borders or in containers. Grow a couple of pots of basil and coriander on a sunny windowsill. Fill your patio or balcony with tomato plants or chillies.

Eating something you've grown yourself is not only satisfying but it also saves money – especially with plants that keep growing back year after year.

If you truly lack a green thumb, you're in good company – I myself am not a natural gardener. I suggest starting with your favourite herb, whatever you cook with most often. A pot of rosemary or thyme can live year round, and those little bundles of dried and fresh herbs are so pricey!

#55
ROTATE YOUR CHOICES

Be flexible. Once you have your meal plan and recipes decided, you head to the shops to load up on ingredients – then you discover there's no marrow anywhere to be had! Instead of ditching the recipe and making something else, be flexible. Here's how.

- Opt for a similar fruit or vegetable when the one you want isn't available or is too costly for you. Use courgettes in place of aubergines, or yellow bell peppers in place of red ones.

- Skip herbs and spices if you don't have them. If possible, substitute a similar one you already have. For example, swap thyme for rosemary.

- No Puy lentils in stock today? Opt for regular green ones.

- I know I told you to follow recipes to the letter, but this is assuming that you're not making a dish for the very first time, and that any of these swaps won't make or break your dish. If you're not confident, skip this tip for now!

#56

OPT FOR FROZEN INSTEAD OF FRESH

Frozen foods have come a long way, and research now shows that some frozen foods may be slightly more nutritious than their fresh counterparts. That's because frozen foods are picked at peak freshness then flash frozen, whereas fresh foods might sit on shelves, lorries or in the fields until past their nutritional and taste prime.

- Frozen broccoli and cauliflower are two of my favourites – cooking them saves time and money, and encourages me to eat more of these veg.

- Frozen tropical fruit is such a luxury – it's sweet and delicious, and you don't have to do any of the work to peel and process it!

- Beyond peas, carrots, green beans and corn – all the basics – look for frozen mushrooms and artichoke hearts.

- Skip any pre-seasoned or flavoured frozen vegetables, and stick with those containing one ingredient: vegetables!

#57

EAT AT HOME

Although it might take a while to break your takeaway habit, your bank account will instantly breathe a sigh of relief. But cooking at home is not only more affordable, it also allows you to be in control of what you eat – restaurant food often contains hidden sugar and salt.

- Set a goal to learn a homemade version of a takeaway favourite once a month. Cook with a friend or your partner and make it a social event.

- Pizza is a manageable place to start and it certainly seems to be universally liked. Yeasted doughs are simple but do require time, then you can top your crust with all your favourite meat-free options. If you crave pepperoni, use olives for the salty richness, then season with fennel, chilli flakes and oregano.

- As you start to eat less meat and more vegetables, you might find your palate shifting. Often I find restaurant food to be too rich and heavy and too skimpy on vegetables. I actually prefer to eat my own food more often than not!

SAVE SCRAPS FOR VEGGIE BROTH

This trick makes me feel so clever and thrifty each time I make a batch of vegetable broth! Stock or broth can be used instead of water to add extra flavour to any savoury dish. I use it in place of water when cooking rice, to loosen up sauces or deglaze a pan, and in soups, of course.

To make your own, simply save all the bits of vegetables you'd normally discard (or, hopefully, compost). I always include onion skins, carrot peelings, celery leaves and mushroom stems, along with garlic and herb stems (like rosemary and thyme). (Avoid any vegetables that are too pungent, like asparagus, cabbage and tomatoes, as well as any that have spoiled.)

Store your scraps in a bag in the freezer. Once the bag is full, place in a pot, cover with water (use equal volumes of vegetables and water), and simmer for an hour or longer. (You can also slow cook it overnight.) Season to taste, strain and store in jars in the fridge for up to two weeks.

#59
DON'T SHOP HUNGRY!

This rule applies no matter what diet you follow. If you go to the supermarket hungry, you will fill your basket with all sorts of things you'll regret later. Convenience foods will seem that much more convenient. Crisps became even more irresistible. And that ice cream seems to be calling your name, too. If you're new to a meat-free diet and find yourself fighting cravings, definitely strategize your shopping trips so you're not famished. You may find yourself in front of the sausage display, willing your resolve to stay strong in the face of temptation.

Shop with an empty stomach, and you'll end up with an empty wallet, too, according to research from the University of Southern California. Researchers found hungry shoppers spent up to 60 per cent more, and sometimes bought non-food items, too. I can tell you from experience that my shopping list becomes optional when my belly rumbles!

EAT WHAT YOU LIKE, AND DON'T SWEAT IT

Don't fall prey to the belief that eating a plant-based diet means eating microgreens, only the rarest of wild mushrooms and the most exclusive organic, cold-pressed olive oils. If you have the means and desire to eat such things, go for it. But a healthy, meat-free diet doesn't need to have all those bells and whistles. Keep your diet simple and heed the words of food activist and journalist Michael Pollan: "Eat food, not too much, mostly plants." I'll edit this sage quote to advise "all plants" versus mostly, but I agree with his sentiments.

A meat-free diet should be free from stress and guilt – you don't have to eat kale if you don't like it. You can bypass the goji berries for plain old raisins. And you have my permission to never eat quinoa instead of good old rice if that's what you prefer. Stick with what you like and what you can afford!

GOING OUT

Being meat free doesn't mean you have to live an ascetic and lonely life. Thankfully, with so many people abstaining from meat, restaurants – from tiny neighbourhood cafés to global chains – are starting to get it. You can find vegetarian and even vegan offerings almost anywhere. From packed lunches to dining out and diverse social settings, I'll walk you through every possible scenario where you might need to consider your dietary preferences.

#61

EAT LEFTOVERS FOR LUNCH

My number one tip, not only for eating a meat-free diet but also for eating more healthily in general, is to pack your lunch. It takes almost no extra time to cook enough for you (and your partner) to take a serving of tonight's supper for tomorrow's lunch. "Tomorrow you" will thank "last night you," and you'll save money and calories. When I gave up meat, I realized how much money I wasted on overpriced, sub-par sandwiches, soups and other lunch fare.

For several years, I worked in a virtual food desert. I didn't have the luxury of tasty lunch options, so I had no choice but to eat the healthy foods I'd packed. I would purposely pack a piece of fruit or raw vegetables as an afternoon snack, too.

If you want to treat yourself and socialize with colleagues at lunch now and again, choose one of the veggie-friendly options on the next few pages.

#62
STICK TO THE APPETIZERS SECTION

Restaurants seem to be much better at offering meat-free sides and starters than main dishes. Use this to your advantage and order a couple of small plates if there are no main courses available without meat. This tactic often saves money, which is a win-win! While it can feel frustrating to not be able to order whatever you want from a menu, or to need to cobble together disparate foods, don't worry about it. It's one meal, so make it an experience. Have back-to-back salad courses. Enjoy a trio of veg and wholegrain sides as a meal. If you're really scraping bottom on a menu, use it as an excuse to have a cocktail and load up on good bread or fries! I've eaten plenty of odd meals since giving up meat and, oftentimes, the strangeness of my choices – frequently the only meat-free offerings – has led to some meaningful discussions about why I choose to eat plants.

#63

ASK FOR SPECIAL TREATMENT

My husband, Sam, is also a vegan and he gets especially riled up when a restaurant leaves the meat out of a dish but adds nothing in its place – or doesn't offer a discount. Most restaurants will happily leave off meat, fish or poultry, and they'll drop some money from your bill, too, since these are the priciest ingredients. Don't be shy about asking if they don't volunteer – it may be the first time someone has posed such a question.

Independent restaurants might have fewer meat-free options on the menu, but they also tend to have more latitude for creativity. If there's nothing on the menu, ask whether the chef is able to create a meat-free dish for you. I've found that, as long as I ask nicely, many chefs jump at the chance to show off their improv skills.

#64

EXPAND YOUR PALATE

I'm American and, as you might know, the land of burgers and steaks is not exactly veggie-friendly. When I gave up meat, I started eating mostly ethnic cuisines, which lend themselves to meat-free eating more than American fare or even British traditional dishes do. Steakhouses, BBQ joints, fish or fried chicken restaurants and Brazilian churrascarias are obviously going to be harder to navigate as a plant-based eater than somewhere with a more diverse menu. If you find yourself at one of these meat-centric restaurants, you won't go hungry – you'll just have to be creative. Ask for steamed or grilled vegetables (enquire whether they're cooked on the same grill as meat), a jacket potato or fries, or salads. Steakhouses tend to have quite lavish sides, so you might encounter something decadently meat-free, like truffle risotto!

#65
KNOW YOUR MEAT-FREE INDIAN OPTIONS

Indian cuisine is often naturally meat-free, especially southern Indian dishes. When dining out with a group, I almost always suggest Indian, as there's something for everyone. The generously spiced curries come in countless plant-based varieties and I leave feeling satisfied – never like I missed out because I don't eat meat.

- Enquire whether dairy – especially cream and ghee – is used in rice and breads if you're vegan.

- Naan is often made with ghee or yogurt, while wholewheat roti tends to be vegan-friendly.

- Opt for any number of legume- and veggie-based soups and stews, like chana masala, baingan bharta and dal. Many use coconut milk in place of cream and some restaurants can easily swap dairy cream for coconut in other dishes.

- Load up on flavourful chutneys – they're meat free and usually dairy free!

- Bonus: the vibrant herbs and spices in Indian food are packed with phytochemicals that support health and well-being and are usually dairy free!

GO BEYOND SUSHI AT JAPANESE RESTAURANTS

Sushi was the last animal product that I gave up, but I soon realized there were numerous fish and meat-free options in Japanese cuisine. When katsu and many ramens are off the menu, you may begin to notice the delectable variety of pickled, sautéed and braised vegetable dishes.

- Cucumber, avocado and pickled vegetable rolls are tasty veg options. Some sushi chefs may be able to accommodate special fish-free rolls.

- Many noodles are made with eggs, so ask if vegan options are available. Soba and udon noodles are traditionally free of eggs.

- Dashi is a stock made with dried fish flakes and the seaweed kombu. Ask whether a vegetable or miso stock could be swapped in.

- Tempura vegetables and skewered vegetables, plus rice and miso broth or salad make for a satisfying, simple meal that's free of meat.

- Look for mushroom or tofu hotpots, as well as dishes made with kabocha squash.

#67

KNOW HOW TO ORDER MEAT-FREE MEXICAN FOOD

Tortilla chips and salsa are meat free, but thankfully your plant-based options don't stop there. With a heavy emphasis on beans, Mexican cuisine is another veggie-friendly staple. However, some beans are cooked with lard or meat, so always ask. Once you've sorted out whether beans (or anything else, like tortillas) contain lard, it's rather simple to eat a meat-free Mexican meal.

- Vegetable, mushroom and bean fajitas, enchiladas (with or without cheese, depending on your diet) and tacos are favourite choices.

- At some authentic restaurants, you might find offerings like nopales (cactus) and huitlacoche (corn smut, a type of fungus that's a delicacy).

- Soups tend to be made with chicken stock or sometimes pork, so ask first.

- When in doubt, ask for more guac! Avocados offer rich creaminess to replace dairy and they're my favourite thing about Mexican food.

- Even if you aren't vegan, consider cutting back on or skipping the cheese and sour cream – they're heavy and often overpower the rest of a dish.

HAVE YOUR PICK OF MIDDLE EASTERN FLAVOURS

While the cultures of the Middle East are quite diverse, the cuisines in the region have in common that they can easily be meat free. With a heavy emphasis on legumes, fresh and grilled or roasted vegetables, olives and olive oil, you will be able to find plenty of veggie-friendly meals and snacks.

- Build a meze platter, with hummus and other veg- or legume-based dips, vegetables, olives, flatbreads and salads.

- Falafel are just one of many legume options. Try braised white beans in tomato sauce, fava beans and chickpeas in any number of preparations or lentil soups (enquire whether vegetable or meat stock was used).

- Bulgur and other wholegrains are a hearty addition to any salad. Tabbouleh is a delicious, filling choice.

- Check to see whether tahini sauce contains dairy, then drizzle the rich, bitter sesame sauce over salads and grilled vegetables.

- To boost my veg intake and not overdo it on pitta and other yummy breads, I often use lettuce or crudités to scoop hummus and other dips.

EXPAND YOUR ITALIAN

Once you venture beyond all the parmesan, meatballs and Bolognese sauce, Italian restaurants are a safe bet for meat-free eaters. (Homemade pasta often contains eggs, so do enquire about that to start.) You'll find endless pasta shapes and options – just ask for those without meat stock, cream or cheese. You can't go wrong with marinara or pomodoro sauce!

- Opt for tomato and olive oil bases for pastas and pizzas over creamy ones.

- Traditional pizzas are delightful without cheese, often highlighting a single ingredient.

- Thick, doughy focaccia is another favourite, albeit carb-heavy, option. Some favourites are olive, onion and rosemary.

- Seek out sides and salads featuring tomatoes, peppers, aubergines and courgettes.

- Depending on the regional influence, some restaurants may feature bean dishes. Enquire whether any use meat, as they often require long cooking and can't be customized.

TAKE ON THAI

Spicy curries, crunchy veg-filled rolls and heaps of thin rice noodles – Thai food is heavy on the vegetables and easily customized to suit your meat-free palate.

- Curry sauces may be prepared in larger batches, using fish sauce. Enquire whether fish products are used in any sauces or dressings.

- Tofu is almost always available at Thai restaurants. While frying it isn't the healthiest preparation, it allows the tofu to soak up the tasty sauces. If you prefer, ask for steamed or marinated tofu instead.

- Pad Thai can be made meat-free, but it usually does contain egg as well, so customize your order as needed.

- Vegetable rolls wrapped in rice paper are a wonderful vegan option and you may also encounter fried veg spring rolls, too. (Double-check that the sauce is fish-free!)

- Tom yum – a spicy, citrus-laden soup – and tom kha – a similar soup that's richer, due to added coconut milk – may contain fish sauce.

#71

KNOW THE SNEAKY PLACES YOU'LL ENCOUNTER MEAT

It's easy to figure out that you'll need to ask for no chicken on a Caesar salad. But did you also know there's (usually) anchovy in the dressing? Depending on your personal beliefs and where you are in your journey, you can decide how strict you want to be and how many questions you want to ask. But, since knowledge is power, you should know where animal products might be lurking in your food.

- **Broth:** Surprisingly, vegetable soups are often made with meat broths, so I always ask. Broth is also used in mashed potatoes, sauces and grains, including risotto.

- **Gelatine:** Aspic, gummy candies and marshmallows all contain gelatine, which comes from the bones and connective tissues of animals.

- **Fish or oyster sauce:** These umami-rich sauces sneak into all kinds of foods – marinades, sauces, curries, etc.

- **Anchovies:** These tiny little fish melt down and become invisible. You'll find them in Worcestershire sauce (though vegan versions exist), Caesar dressing, marinades and pasta sauces.

ASK QUESTIONS AND DON'T APOLOGIZE

I am not one who enjoys confrontation or debate, so asking tough questions of kind restaurant staff made me uncomfortable when I first gave up meat. However, I found that if I approached the situation with a positive attitude and kindness, most were willing to provide me with the answers I needed. In the last few years, more restaurants list vegan or vegetarian items on their menu and some have an entirely separate menu!

You may encounter waiting staff or chefs who won't know what "vegan" means, or they think meat-free means you still eat poultry or fish. If you do, offer a brief explanation, be clear with your questions and don't feel the need to apologize. Regardless of your reason to exclude meat from your diet, it's your right to do so. Your questions are a minor inconvenience.

#73

BRING A DISH TO A PARTY

Though hosts usually insist we shouldn't bring anything but ourselves to a party, that's just politesse. Most hosts would actually be thrilled if you brought something. I always offer to bring a meat-free dish, especially when the host isn't a close friend or if they don't know much about meat-free eating. This ensures you have something to eat if the host forgets or doesn't know you don't eat meat. I've found that, even in groups where bringing food to a party seems a bit of a faux pas, my sans-meat option always disappears. If you find there are few vegan offerings, eat what you can, discreetly enquire about ingredients and – when all else fails – load up on bread.

Better yet, host a meat-free dinner party. I love having friends to dinner to show them the delicious diversity of vegan foods.

#74

DIY MEALS ARE YOUR BFF

You're likely not the only person with dietary restrictions in your group of friends or family. You may have a friend who's gluten-free, one who's allergic to soya, or a sister who can't stand coriander. When you're hosting a group or planning an event, customizable meals are the way to please all palates. Try taco bars, roll-your-own sushi, or personalized pizzas. That way, you don't have to keep track of who eats – or doesn't eat – certain things.

In families or settings where not everyone is meat free, remember that it's easier to add than to subtract. If someone must have meat, cook it separately and keep it to the side. Use vegetable broth and olive oil instead of chicken or beef stock and butter. Keep cheese on the side, too. Starting with a plant-based meal helps you pack in more nutrients (usually) and ensures everyone gets to fill their plate.

#75

SNEAK IN YOUR OWN FOOD

Please don't take a packed lunch to a restaurant, but if you know there will be few (or no) meat-free options, break the rules and bring some food. I've taken trail mix to a football match, packed a peanut butter sandwich and fruit for an afternoon at an amusement park and taken a cooler with plant-based food along to the beach. When there's no choice between eating meat or going hungry, provide for yourself.

At events where it would be socially awkward to bring food, I've been known to sneak away if there is no other option. Once, at a friend's wedding, my husband and I stole off for a quick bite when we realized there were no vegan options for us – and had a long night of dancing and drinking ahead. We ordered and ate as quickly as we could, then hurried back before the dinner plates had been cleared.

KNOW HOW TO BULK UP MEAGRE MEAT-FREE DISHES

There's a lingering myth that meat-free eaters don't like to eat. Au contraire! We expect the same quality and diversity of ingredients as omnivores. So when you see that a restaurant has tried (but fallen short), get creative. It's been rare that I've had to use these "hacks", but it's nice to have them in mind in case you need them.

- Ask for a side of beans, nuts or seeds to accompany a skimpy salad.

- If you're holding the cheese, request avocado or extra sauce or dressing in its place.

- Double up on sides like pulses or rice.

- Order olives or grilled vegetables to make boring pasta with red sauce more flavourful.

- When served steamed vegetables and rice (why do restaurants think meat-free equals restrictive?), add flavour with lime or lemon wedges or balsamic vinegar. Salad dressings are good on plain vegetables, too.

#77

FOR EVENTS BEYOND YOUR CONTROL, PLANNING IS KEY

It's easy enough to influence restaurant choice when you're planning a Friday-night dinner with friends, but when you're required to attend a business luncheon or a week-long conference off site, meat-free options might not be readily available.

When you have some notice, call ahead to restaurants and hotels to enquire whether special arrangements could be made. Most can accommodate with enough notice. If you're caught off-guard at a luncheon, snag the attention of a server and ask that the protein be left off your plate.

And always keep a snack on hand. I never leave home without a small container of nuts or a granola bar in my handbag. It's not haute cuisine, but it will work at a pinch.

I assert myself in social settings when my eating choices are challenged, but I also believe that someone else's big day or a work event is not the time to start a conversation about being vegan (unless asked directly).

DO YOUR HOMEWORK

If you're not a finicky eater and will happily eat anything, as long as it's meat free, you don't need to plan ahead every time you eat away from home. If you're a foodie, some planning can prevent disappointing meals.

- Peruse online menus. I usually check out the menu before committing to a new restaurant, to ensure they have options I'll like.

- Seek recommendations on Facebook. The hive mind of social media is quite useful for soliciting restaurant tips, and if you're in a new city, you may find somewhere off the beaten path that tourists rarely frequent.

- Use apps like Happy Cow and Yelp. Happy Cow's website and app can help you find veggie-friendly restaurants, grocery stores and other businesses around the world. Yelp reviews can be filtered by keyword and you can often get a sense of how diners with special requests are treated by reading a few reviews.

FIND A MEETUP GROUP
FOR SUPPORT

Beyond restaurant suggestions, Facebook's community has been a wonderful resource for my meat-free journey. Seek out groups in your area – many have real-life meetups at veg-friendly venues. And if you're shy about meeting folks you met online, use the groups for support when you face uncomfortable situations (my manager berated me for not eating the lamb at a company dinner) or to share your own favourite meals and restaurants.

My friend, Lisa, owns a vegan brewery and runs an animal rescue – and she started a fun Facebook group for vegans, vegetarians and the veg-curious among us. We share news stories about the meat-free movement, recipes we want to try, and tips on saving money and dining out when you don't eat meat. You might search for a group of young vegans in your area, or one for meat-free pensioners on a budget. You're not in this alone!

KEEP AN OPEN MIND

I've occasionally been harassed or mocked for my meat-free preferences, but most people are fascinated by it and want to know more. I focus on the positives – the health benefits and variety of delicious foods I can eat. Once they see what you can and do eat without meat, it often piques their interest. I try to stay open and assume the best in people – change is hard to accept and when you challenge someone's idea of normal, they often close down or respond defensively.

So, when the chef at an Italian restaurant scoffs at your request for no Parmesan or no meat stock in a dish – or when your sister criticizes your questioning of restaurant staff – take a deep breath. You can't control their reaction. You can control your own. Stay positive and firm – you have the right to choose what foods you do and don't eat.

GETTING CREATIVE

If you're used to including fish and meat in every meal, you might feel like something's missing on the plate – but not to worry. This final chapter of the book has ways of getting creative with vegetarian and vegan ingredients. When you feel tempted, remember giving up meat and dairy is the "single biggest way" you can reduce your environmental impact!

#81
LEARN TO COOK

This might sound somewhat silly, but you'll need to learn how to cook if you want to eat a healthy, meat-free diet. Sure, you can rely on prepared foods and takeaway but that's not sustainable or affordable. As a foodie, at first I worried that giving up meat meant losing my passion for cooking. I didn't yet understand how diverse the plant-based cooking world could be! I became adventurous, seeking out cuisines that were naturally plant free, experimenting with new-to-me herbs and spices and getting familiar with how to cook tofu and tempeh.

If you currently don't cook much, that's OK. Pick up a meat-free cookbook aimed at beginners – I like any of Isa Chandra Moskowitz's titles, *Vegan Planet* by Robin Robertson, *Vegetarian Cooking for Everyone* by Deborah Madison or *How to Cook Anything Vegetarian* by Mark Bittman. Though I am now vegan, I still refer to these latter two cookbooks often. Then, pick a recipe and start cooking.

DON'T FEAR THE KNIFE

While we are taught to fear and respect sharp knives, dull ones are more dangerous. Here are some basic tips:

- Keep your knives sharp and always know where your fingers are.

- Keep your eye on the knife and tuck your fingertips under to keep from slicing them off.

- Buy a medium-size chef's knife, along with a paring knife and a serrated one.

- Watch YouTube videos or take a course in basic knife skills if you're not comfortable with terms like chop, dice or mince.

- If you can learn to chop or dice an onion, slice a pepper and mince garlic, you're well on your way to creating delicious dishes. Once you've mastered those three, move on to cuts like julienne, batonnet or chiffonade.

- Tip: When slicing unruly or round vegetables or fruit, start by establishing a flat edge to avoid rolling. Take a thin slice off one side of a carrot or halve a potato, for example.

#83

BE GENEROUS WITH HERBS AND SPICES

Herbs and spices not only add loads of flavour – with virtually no calories, salt or fat – but they are also a concentrated source of phytochemicals, valuable nutrients found only in plants. Get comfortable with them in the kitchen:

- Dried herbs have a shelf life of a few months.

- When a recipe specifies fresh herbs, but you have only dried (or vice versa), it's usually OK to swap them.

- Use three times the amount of fresh herbs as dried, which are more concentrated and potent.

- Cook dried herbs to release their flavour and, for good measure, give them a good rub between your hands first to release more of their volatile oils and other compounds.

- Add dried herbs and spices to the pot when you cook aromatics like onions or shallots, allowing the oil to help unlock more of their flavour. (This is called "blooming".)

- Fresh herbs are used for garnish and often added at the end of cooking.

#84

BEANS ARE YOUR BEST FRIEND

Lentils, beans and other pulses are so affordable and nutritious! I eat them daily, in soups and stews, blended into dips and sauces and even added to sweets and smoothies. Here are some inventive ways to use them:

White beans: These creamy, soft beans are perfect braised in tomato-based dishes, blended in place of heavy cream for white sauces and pureed with fresh herbs and lemon juice for a simple dip for crudités.

Black beans: In addition to being one of my favourite savoury beans, black beans are – believe it or not – a secret ingredient in healthier, cheaper baked goods. Puree them into cakes, brownies and bars (in place of some of the oil or eggs).

To cook dried beans: Soak in water overnight, then rinse and cover with 2.5 cm (1 in) of water. Add a 2.5 cm (1 in) square of kombu (seaweed) to improve digestibility. Simmer until soft and season to taste, then proceed with your recipe.

#85

MIND YOUR MOTHER (SAUCES)

Classic French cooking bases most sauces on one of five "mother" sauces – none of which is vegan. However, you can remove the meat, eggs and dairy from them all rather easily.

Most start with a roux, or a mix of butter and flour to thicken the sauce. However, you can use either oil or vegan butter to achieve the same results. From there, here's how to make the mother sauces plant based to create endless tasty meals:

Béchamel: A white sauce made from a roux and milk. Substitute an unsweetened non-dairy milk, like soya or oat.

Velouté: Made from roux and a light-coloured stock. Use veggie broth instead of chicken stock.

Espagnole: Made from roux and a darker stock, like beef. Substitute mushroom broth.

Tomato: Made from roux and pureed tomatoes. It's already meat free, and it's vegan without the butter in the roux.

Hollandaise: Typically made from egg yolks, butter and lemon juice or wine. I cheat and add extra lemon juice and olive oil to my cashew cream sauce (see p.38).

#86

SOAK UP THE FLAVOUR

Marinades aren't just for meat. Tofu, tempeh, seitan, mushrooms and vegetables all taste delicious when marinated. You can use your favourite meat marinades (being mindful of hidden fish sauce) or try a new one.

This is my go-to everyday marinade: 1 tablespoon each of red miso, vegan Worcestershire sauce, Dijon mustard, sugar, apple cider vinegar, balsamic vinegar and olive oil, plus ¼ teaspoon of black pepper and ½ teaspoon of dried thyme or rosemary. Toss and refrigerate for up to four hours, then cook as desired.

For a Korean-inspired marinade: 1 teaspoon each of soy sauce and sesame seeds, plus 2 minced garlic cloves and 2 tablespoons each of Korean red pepper flakes, rice vinegar, brown sugar and toasted sesame oil.

#87

STRATEGIZE YOUR SALT USE

Table salt is fine if that's what you have, but I like salty ingredients to do double duty, imparting richness and umami or texture as well as salinity.

Olives and capers: Chop a spoonful to stretch their flavour. Sprinkle on top of salads, pasta or hummus.

Soy sauce: The varieties are seemingly endless – tamari, shoyu, dark and light soy sauce are some of the more common varieties. Add to Asian-inspired meals, stir into marinades or sprinkle over steamed vegetables or tofu.

Miso paste: This traditional Japanese ingredient is made from fermented soybeans or other legumes. So as not to destroy the delicate probiotics, stir this in at the end of cooking. White miso is used for soup, while richer, dark red miso is for marinades, stews and glazes.

Vegemite or Marmite: These yeasty pastes are good on more than toast! They're the secret ingredient in my homemade three-bean chilli and they add a layer of complexity to any dish or sauce. Spread a thin layer on toast, then add mashed avocado!

Preserved lemons: Commonly used in Moroccan cuisine, these salt-packed lemons add a tartness that's a delightful finishing ingredient. I love mincing a segment of preserved lemon – a little goes a long way – then adding to guacamole or hummus.

#88

ROAST YOUR NUTS

I prefer to buy nuts and seeds raw and whole when possible, to keep them fresher, longer. I use raw nuts to make milks and sauces, but I like to roast or toast them to intensify their flavour in dishes. Spread them in a single layer on a baking sheet and roast for 10 minutes (or until fragrant) at 180°C (350°F, gas 4). Transfer to another dish to cool, as carry-over heat may cause them to burn.

Toasting nuts amplifies their nuttiness. Chop them to spread the flavour throughout a dish and season to taste as desired. In addition to salt (or soy sauce, added before roasting) and pepper, try curry powder, smoked paprika or cinnamon.

Roasted nuts make a great snack on their own, or I use them atop grain bowls, salads or in veggie burgers.

#89

BEHOLD THE MIGHTY AVOCADO

When I gave up cheese and meat, I started eating a lot of avocados. They contain heart-healthy fats and fibre, and I just really like their creaminess. In addition to the now ubiquitous avocado toast and classic guacamole, I use avocados in:

Salad dressings: Use in place of oil in a traditional vinaigrette, or blend with plenty of lime juice, coriander, green onions and salt for a guacamole-inspired dressing. Use it anywhere you'd normally use mayonnaise.

Desserts: Blend avocado with coconut milk and dark cocoa powder for a decadent dessert that no one will know doesn't contain cream! (Sweeten with maple syrup, if desired.)

Soup: Blend an avocado with a cucumber, half a jalapeño (optional), a handful of coriander or basil leaves, plus lemon juice and salt to taste. Thin with water as desired for a cool summer soup.

#90
COOK YOUR TOMATO PURÉE

Pop quiz: Do you simply plop tomato purée into a pot of soup or pasta sauce? You're not using it to its full potential – and it might add a tinny or raw tomato flavour rather than tasty richness. Instead, add it once you've softened your aromatics, allowing it to cook. It will stick to the bottom of the pan and turn brown (see the next tip to learn how not to waste those tasty bits), so stir often.

Once it's fragrant and darker in colour, you can proceed with your recipe, stirring other ingredients so they are coated in all that tomatoey goodness. Rich in umami, tomato purée caramelizes when you cook it, and it adds the same sweetness and intensity that sundried tomatoes do. (Those are another wonderful, umami-rich ingredient that I use in soups, stews and anywhere I need more heft.)

#91
DEGLAZE YOUR PAN

The bits that stick to the bottom of the pan are tiny little flavour bombs, so don't waste them. Anytime an ingredient gets some colour and deposits brown stickiness in the pan, that's called fond (French for crust). Reintegrate that deliciousness into your dish using a classic technique called deglazing.

Start by adding a liquid to the pot or pan – a few tablespoons will do. Though you can use water, it won't add any extra flavour. Instead opt for wine, dry sherry or vegetable broth. As soon as you add the liquid, scrape the bottom of the pan vigorously with a wooden spoon to lift the fond. If the recipe calls for more liquid, add it after most of the deglazing liquid has evaporated.

I especially love using this technique with mushrooms, then using the fond to create a pan sauce that no one will know is meat free!

#92
GET SAUCY

Since vegetables, wholegrains and – when cooked simply – ingredients like tofu and tempeh lack fat, your basic meals might feel like they are missing something at first. Compensate by adding a sauce – any kind that you prefer. Sauces impart flavour and turn a simple dish into something special.

Start with the mother sauces explained in this chapter, then get creative. Stir in fresh herbs, extra citrus, or your favourite spice (like cumin, smoked paprika or curry).

I like to use fresh herbs or greens as the basis for fresh, light sauces. Try parsley-based chimichurri from Argentina, the similar Italian version called salsa verde (with added capers), any type of pesto (beyond basil, try parsley, rocket or coriander) or Moroccan chermoula with coriander, parsley and mint.

#93

FINISH WITH AN ACID

If you are trained to reach for salt at the table or when finishing a dish, pause before you start shaking it on. Our taste buds love contrast, and a chef's secret is reaching for an acid instead of salt.

Salt your food as you go along, but when you taste it for the last time before serving, notice whether it is flat on the palate. If so, try one of these acidic ingredients:

- Lemon, lime or orange juice
- Wine (be sure to cook off the alcohol)
- Vinegar – especially sherry, balsamic or a flavoured variety

These acids give foods the "zing" your taste buds crave. When foods are overly creamy, rich or dull, your palate needs something to keep its interest. Sometimes a simple squeeze of a lime wedge is just the trick!

CHANGE YOUR LIFE
WITH CASHEWS

Blending with water, a salty ingredient and an acid transforms raw cashews from a bland nut into the creamiest, most delicious sauces and dairy stand-ins. Once I discovered the magic of cashews, I never once missed dairy. Here's how to get started:

Soak 125 g (4.5 oz) of raw, unsalted cashews in hot water for a few hours. Drain, then blend with 125 ml (4.5 fl oz) of water until creamy. Add 1 tablespoon of lemon juice, and salt or white miso paste to taste Then you can customize in infinite ways:

- Add another 75 ml (2.5 fl oz) of water for a béchamel sauce.
- Reduce water by 50 ml (2 fl oz) for a thick, cheese-like spread.
- Stir in chopped fresh herbs, or blend in 1 clove of garlic.
- Add more lemon juice for a hollandaise sauce, plus fresh or dried tarragon for béarnaise.
- Blend in roasted red peppers, sundried tomatoes or tomato purée, then simmer and serve over pasta.
- Stir in prepared dairy-free pesto.
- Blend in 125 g (4.5 oz) of steamed cauliflower or butternut squash for a lighter cream sauce.
- Add nutritional yeast for a cheesier sauce for pasta.

#95

GO BEYOND HUMMUS

While I'll never turn down a good traditional hummus (with extra tahini, preferably), I also like to create different bean dips. They're delicious with crudités or crackers, spread thickly on toast, or as a sandwich or wrap spread. Bean dip is incredibly easy and affordable. Here is my basic recipe, along with some variations:

Start with 1 x 400 g (14 oz) tin of beans, drained and rinsed well. Add to a food processor or blender with 1 clove of garlic or 1 chopped spring onion, the juice of a lemon, a tablespoon of olive oil and salt to taste. Blend until completely smooth, adding water as desired to reach a consistency you like. From there, customize it:

- Blend white beans with fresh herbs – try basil or tarragon in summer, rosemary and thyme in winter.
- Purée with a roasted red pepper, roasted carrots or sundried tomatoes. This works with black or white beans.
- Create edamame hummus with a bit of grated ginger, optional wasabi to taste, soy sauce instead of salt and toasted sesame oil in place of olive oil.
- Blend black bean dip with spicy salsa and sprinkle nutritional yeast on top. Serve warm.

LEARN TO MAKE VEGGIE BURGERS

Save money and use up odds and ends in the fridge by making veggie burgers. Here is my formula, which you can change up by swapping herbs and spices, types of beans and vegetables, etc.

RECIPE:

To make eight burgers, start by sautéing half an onion, diced, with about 250 g (9 oz) shredded vegetables (courgettes, beetroot, carrots, etc.) and 1 tablespoon of your seasoning of choice.

Add 1 tablespoon of tomato purée, cooking until fragrant, then deglaze the pan with a tablespoon of vinegar. Cook until there is no excess water in the pan. Transfer to a food processor with 1 tin of beans, drained and rinsed, along with 200 g (7 oz) of cooked rice or another whole grain. Pulse until mostly mixed, then season with salt and pepper. Wet your hands, then shape the mixture into eight patties. Place on a baking sheet lined with baking paper, and bake at 200°C (390°F, gas 6) for 45 minutes, flipping halfway. Let cool for 15 minutes before serving.

#97
SCRAMBLE TOFU FOR BREAKFAST

Tofu scramble is my favourite savoury breakfast, and I make it every week. It has replaced eggs in my repertoire of meals. Here is my basic recipe, to which you can add any vegetables you'd like.

Heat a large pan over medium-high heat and add 1 tablespoon of oil. Add 1 small yellow onion, diced, and a few chopped mushrooms if desired. Cook, stirring often, until softened, then add 450 g (16 oz) of firm tofu, crumbled.

Season with: 1 teaspoon each of ground cumin, yellow curry powder and turmeric, plus half a teaspoon of dried ground thyme or rosemary and paprika. Reduce the heat to medium-low. Cook, stirring often, for about 15 minutes, until the tofu starts to brown and is no longer watery. Stir in plenty of nutritional yeast, salt and pepper. Serve with avocado toast or roasted potatoes.

EMBRACE THE BOWL MEAL

You do not need to reinvent the wheel every night. Keep your meals simple. At my house, we often eat what I refer to as "bowl meals". I start with a base of steamed vegetables, add a serving of wholegrains or roasted root vegetables and top with beans, tofu or tempeh. Finally, we add a sauce and fun toppings like seeds or chopped nuts, avocado, fermented vegetables, sprouts, etc.

Using this formula, you can mix and match simple ingredients to create delicious meals without spending the whole night in the kitchen. Here are some favourites:

- Roasted sweet potatoes with steamed spring greens, black beans, salsa and diced red onions.

- Brown rice with broccoli and tofu, plus a soy-ginger sauce and coriander leaves.

- Whole grain pasta with red lentils and sautéed red peppers, topped with creamy cashew sauce and fresh parsley.

- Bulgur wheat with chickpeas, raw kale, tahini sauce, spring onions and sliced radishes.

#99

MASTER THE SHEET-PAN DINNER

Another fun, simple way to construct your meals is with the "baking tray dinner". You simply place all your ingredients on a baking tray and bake them together. Dinner is ready without dirtying a whole load of dishes.

Start by preheating the oven to 200°C (390°F, gas 6). Line a baking sheet with baking paper. For four servings you need 500 g (18 oz) of assorted vegetables, chopped into equal-sized pieces, as well as a tablespoon of oil and a packet of tofu and tempeh, cubed. Sprinkle on your favourite herbs and spices, then spread the ingredients on the baking sheet. Roast for 30 minutes until the tempeh/tofu is starting to brown and the vegetables are soft.

Some of my preferred vegetables to roast are Brussels sprouts, broccoli, cauliflower, peppers, onions, courgettes, sweet potatoes and butternut squash – but let the sky be the limit. You can try asparagus, aubergine or mushrooms, too.

#100

TAKE HELP WHERE YOU CAN

Eating whole, unprocessed foods is always best, but it's nice to have ready-to-eat offerings when life gets busy or you have a hankering for a comfort food. I like to keep one or two frozen meals or tins of soup on hand for times I don't feel like cooking. Here are some brands to look for.

- Amy's Kitchen offers an array of good quality, meat-free meals, many of which are vegan and/or gluten free. Top picks: soups, Mexican cuisine and veggie burgers.

- The Fry Family Food Co. makes a wide array of meat alternatives, from hot dogs and chicken-style strips to battered prawn-style pieces and banger-style traditional sausages.

- Violife makes cheese so good you'll swear it's made from dairy! Try the Just Like Blue Cheese, Mediterranean-Style Block (like halloumi) and the Just Like Provolone.

- When in doubt, visit your local health food store and inquire about new brands worth trying.

FINAL TIP
KEEP TRYING NEW FOODS

Even though I've been meat free since 2006, I am still learning new cooking techniques and trying new foods. Make a goal to buy a new cookbook every couple of months (start a swap with friends to save money) and cook one recipe a week. Shop at different markets – I discovered an Indian foods market in my town, and I've had such fun experimenting with different spices and pulses! Follow meat-free bloggers and Instagram accounts (but don't worry if your meals aren't as photogenic as theirs – it's all about the taste).

Your meat-free life is helping your health, the planet and all furry, finned and feathered inhabitants upon it. Every shopping trip, meal and bite supports the greater good – so keep that in mind when looking for culinary inspiration.

I hope this book provides a strong foundation as you venture out into this brave, new (meat-free) world!

FURTHER READING

INTRODUCTION

https://www.independent.co.uk/life-style/food-and-drink/vegans-uk-rise-popularity-plant-based-diets-veganism-figures-survey-compare-the-market-a8286471.html

http://www.onegreenplanet.org/news/six-percent-of-americans-identify-as-vegan/

HEALTHY LIVING

https://www.theguardian.com/news/2018/mar/01/bacon-cancer-processed-meats-nitrates-nitrites-sausages

https://www.eatrightpro.org/~/media/eatrightpro%20files/practice/position%20and%20practice%20papers/position%20papers/vegetarian-diet.ashx

https://www.nutritionjrnl.com/article/S0899-9007(14)00423-7/abstract

https://link.springer.com/article/10.1007/s11606-015-3390-7

https://www.nutrition.org.uk/nutritionscience/nutrients-food-and-ingredients/dietary-fibre.html

https://academic.oup.com/jn/article/130/2/272S/4686350

https://www.pcrm.org/media/news/vegetarian-diet-is-associated-with-lower-cholesterol-levels-according-to-meta-analysis-in-nutrition

https://heartuk.org.uk/cholesterol-and-diet

https://ods.od.nih.gov/factsheets/Iron-HealthProfessional/

https://www.vegansociety.com/resources/nutrition-and-health/nutrients/vitamin-b12/what-every-vegan-should-know-about-vitamin-b12

https://www.ncbi.nlm.nih.gov/pubmed/16407732

https://www.ncbi.nlm.nih.gov/pubmed/12936959

SURVIVING WITHOUT MEAT

http://www.who.int/features/qa/cancer-red-meat/en/

SAVING MONEY

https://www.tandfonline.com/doi/abs/10.1080/19320248.2015.1045675?journalCode=when20

https://www.vegsoc.org/sslpage.aspx?pid=525

http://www.fao.org/save-food/resources/keyfindings/en/

https://www.health.harvard.edu/blog/organic-food-no-more-nutritious-than-conventionally-grown-food-201209055264

https://www.food.gov.uk/business-guidance/pesticides-in-food

https://www.tescoplc.com/news/blogs/topics/wicked-kitchen-derek-sarno-tesco/

https://well.blogs.nytimes.com/2016/11/18/are-frozen-fruits-and-vegetables-as-nutritious-as-fresh/

https://news.usc.edu/78755/are-you-hungry-best-to-eat-first-and-shop-later-study-finds/

GETTING CREATIVE

https://www.theguardian.com/environment/2018/may/31/avoiding-meat-and-dairy-is-single-biggest-way-to-reduce-your-impact-on-earth

STOCKISTS

Online:

www.veganstore.co.uk

    100% vegan store, offering food as well as cosmetics, toiletries, health-care items, and clothing.

shop.thevegankind.com

    100% vegan store, offering food (including chilled foods) and cosmetics, toiletries, health-care items, and clothing.

www.buywholefoodsonline.co.uk

    Good source for bulk foods, including nuts, seeds and herbs.

www.veganonline.com.au

    Vegan food, health and beauty website

www.veganperfection.com.au

    Vegan food and health website, with wholesale orders available

plantgoodness24.ie

    Vegan foods and natural health and home products

Bricks-and-mortar:

www.greenbaysupermarket.co.uk

    London's first vegan Supermarket (online shopping available), based in West Kensington

www.crueltyfreeshop.com.au

    Vegan supermarket chain (online shopping available) with locations in Canberra, Melbourne, Brisbane and Sydney

Le Labo

    Vegan fragrance, candles, grooming products and more with global outlets. Also available online for worldwide shipping.

The Body Shop
    50 per cent of the Body Shop's products are vegan and 100 per cent are vegetarian. Global outlets and online.
Harmless Store
    This London store is plastic-free and zero waste, offering many vegan and vegetarian foods and household items.

Eating out:
UK
Temple of Seitan, London E9 6NA
V Rev, Manchester M4 1HN
Terre à Terre, Brighton BN1 1HQ
Vegetarian Food Studio, Cardiff CF11 6JU
Mono, Glasgow G1 5RB
387 Ormeau Road, Belfast BT7 3GP

USA
Vedge, Philadelphia PA19107
Plant, Asheville NC 28801
Crossroads, Los Angeles CA 90046
The Cinnamon Snail, NY 10121

Australia
Smith & Daughters, Melbourne VIC 3065
The Raw Kitchen, Fremantle WA 6160
Iku Wholefood, various locations

INDEX